Contents

The alkaline diet is based on the theory that the foods you eat change your pH level to either acidic or alkaline. The belief is that consuming a high amount of acidic foods will cause your body harm, whereas eating alkaline or neutral foods can improve your health.

The diet focuses on eating fresh fruits and vegetables (that are considered alkaline) to keep your body at an optimal pH level, which is a measure of acids and alkalis throughout the body using a scale ranging from 0 to 14.

Acidic substances range from 0 to 7; alkaline foods range from 7 to 14. Seven is considered neutral—neither acidic or alkaline. This concept started centuries ago, in the mid-1800s, with the "dietary ash hypothesis"—a theory that once food metabolizes in the body, the particles leave either an acid or alkaline ash.

The 2022 U.S. News and World Report Best Diets ranks the alkaline diet number 30 in Best Diets Overall and gives the diet an overall score of 2.4/5. Its ranking is based on the lack of quality research to support the diet, the many rules that make it difficult to follow, and its ineffectiveness for weight loss. The

Alkaline Diet performed the worst in fast weight loss, overall weight loss, diabetes, and easiness to follow.

Chapter one

There are all types of diets out there — some good, some bad — but there is perhaps no diet better for longevity and staving off disease than a mostly plant-based alkaline diet.

Don't just take my word for it. A 2012 review published in the Journal of Environmental Health found that achieving pH balance by eating an alkaline diet can be helpful in reducing morbidity and mortality from numerous chronic diseases and ailments — such as hypertension, diabetes, arthritis, vitamin D deficiency and low bone density, just to name a few.

How do alkaline diets work? Research shows that diets consisting of highly alkaline foods — fresh vegetables, fruits and unprocessed plant-based sources of protein, for example — result in a more alkaline urine pH level, which helps protect healthy cells and balance essential mineral levels. This can be especially important for women doing intermittent fasting and/or following the keto diet, as hormone levels can be altered.

Alkaline diets (also known as the alkaline ash diets) have been shown to help:

- prevent plaque formation in blood vessels
- stop calcium from accumulating in urine
- prevent kidney stones
- build stronger bones
- reduce muscle wasting or spasms
- and much more

What Is An Alkaline Diet?

An alkaline diet is one that is intended to help balance the blood pH level of the fluids in your body, including your blood and urine.

This diet goes by several different names, including:

- the alkaline ash diet
- alkaline acid diet
- acid ash diet
- pH diet
- Dr. Sebi's alkaline diet (Dr. Sebi was an herbalist who created a plant-based diet version)

Your pH is partially determined by the mineral density of the foods you eat. All living organisms and life forms on Earth depend on maintaining appropriate pH levels, and it's often said that disease and disorder cannot take root in a body that has a balanced pH.

The principles of the acid ash hypothesis help make up the tenets of the alkaline diet. According to research published in Journal of Bone and Mineral Research, "The acid-ash hypothesis posits that protein and grain foods, with a low potassium intake, produce a diet acid load, net acid excretion (NAE), increased urine calcium, and release of calcium from the skeleton, leading to osteoporosis.

The alkaline diet aims to prevent this from happening by carefully taking food pH levels into consideration in an attempt to limit dietary acid intake.

Although some experts might not totally agree with this statement, nearly all agree that human life requires a very tightly controlled pH level of the blood of about 7.365–7.4. As Forbe's Magazine puts it, "Our bodies go to extraordinary lengths to maintain safe pH levels."

Your pH can range between 7.35 to 7.45 depending on the time of day, your diet, what you last ate and when you last went to the bathroom. If you develop electrolyte imbalances and frequently consume too many acidic foods — aka acid ash foods — your body's changing pH level can result in increased "acidosis."

What we call pH is short for the potential of hydrogen. It's a measure of the acidity or alkalinity of the body's fluids and tissues.

It's measured on a scale from 0 to 14. The more acidic a solution is, the lower its pH. The more alkaline, the higher the number is.

A pH of around 7 is considered neutral, but since the optimal human body tends to be around 7.4, we consider the healthiest pH to be one that's slightly alkaline.

These levels also vary throughout the body, with the stomach the most acidic region. Even very tiny alterations in the pH level of various organisms can cause major problems.

For example, due to environmental concerns, such as increasing CO_2 deposition, the pH of the ocean has dropped from 8.2 to 8.1, and various life forms living in the ocean have greatly suffered.

The pH level is also crucial for growing plants, and therefore it greatly affects the mineral content of the foods we eat. Minerals in the ocean, soil and human body are used as buffers to maintain optimal pH levels, so when acidity rises, minerals fall.

Here's some background on acid/alkalinity in the human diet, plus key points about how alkaline diets can be beneficial:

- Researchers believe that when it comes to the total acid load of the human diet, "there have been considerable changes from hunter-gatherer civilizations to the present." Following the agricultural revolution and then mass industrialization of our food supply over the last 200 years, the food we eat has significantly less potassium, magnesium and chloride, along with more sodium, compared to diets of the past.
- Normally, the kidneys maintain our electrolyte levels (those of calcium, magnesium, potassium and sodium). When we're exposed to overly acidic substances, these electrolytes are used to combat acidity.
- According to the Journal of Environmental Health review mentioned earlier, the ratio of potassium to sodium in most people's diets has changed dramatically. Potassium used to outnumber sodium by 10:1, however now the ratio has dropped to 1:3. People eating a "Standard American Diet" now consume three times as much sodium as potassium on

average! This contributes greatly to an alkaline environment in our bodies.

- Many children and adults today consume a high-sodium diet that's very low in not only magnesium and potassium, but also antioxidants, fiber and essential vitamins. On top of that, the typical Western diet is high in refined fats, simple sugars, sodium and chloride.
- All of these changes to the human diet have resulted in increased "metabolic acidosis." In other words, the pH levels of many people's bodies are no longer optimal. On top of this, many are suffering from low nutrient intake and problems such as potassium and magnesium deficiency.

Health Benefits

Why is an alkaline diet good for you? Alkaline foods supply important nutrients that help stop accelerated signs of aging and a gradual loss of organ and cellular functions.

As explained more below, alkaline diet benefits may include helping slow down degeneration of tissues and bone mass, which can be compromised when too much acidity robs us of key minerals.

Protects Bone Density and Muscle Mass

Your intake of minerals plays an important role in the development and maintenance of bone structures. Research suggests that the more alkalizing fruits and vegetables someone eats, the better protection that person might have from experiencing decreased bone strength and muscle wasting as she ages, known as sarcopenia.

An alkaline diet can support bone health by balancing the ratio of minerals that are important for building bones and maintaining lean muscle mass, including calcium, magnesium and phosphate.

The diet may also help improve production of growth hormones and vitamin D absorption, which further protects bones in addition to mitigating many other chronic diseases.

Lowers Risk for Hypertension and Stroke

One of the anti-aging effects of an alkaline diet is that it decreases inflammation and causes an increase in growth hormone production.

This has been shown to improve cardiovascular health and offer protection against common problems like high cholesterol, hypertension (high blood pressure), kidney stones, stroke and even memory loss.

Lowers Chronic Pain and Inflammation

Studies have found a connection between an alkaline diet and reduced levels of chronic pain. Chronic acidosis has been found to contribute to chronic back pain, headaches, muscle spasms, menstrual symptoms, inflammation and joint pain.

One study conducted by the Society for Minerals and Trace Elements in Germany found that when patients with chronic back pain were given an alkaline supplement daily for four weeks, 76 of 82 patients reported significant decreases in pain as measured by the "Arhus low back pain rating scale."

Boosts Vitamin Absorption and Helps Prevent Magnesium Deficiency

An increase in magnesium is required for the function of hundreds of enzyme systems and bodily processes. Many people are deficient in magnesium and as a result experience heart complications, muscle pains, headaches, sleep troubles and anxiety.

Available magnesium is also required to activate vitamin D and prevent vitamin D deficiency, which is important for overall immune and endocrine functioning.

Helps Improve Immune Function and Possibly Cancer Protection

When cells lack enough minerals to properly dispose of waste or oxygenate the body fully, the whole body suffers. Vitamin absorption is compromised by mineral loss, while toxins and pathogens accumulate in the body and weaken the immune system.

Can an alkaline diet help prevent cancer? While the topic is controversial and still unproven, research published in the British Journal of Radiology found evidence that cancerous cell death (apoptosis) was more likely to occur in an alkaline body.

Cancer prevention is believed to be associated with an alkaline shift in pH due to an alteration in electric charges and the release of basic components of proteins. Alkalinity can help decrease inflammation and the risk for diseases like cancer — plus an alkaline diet has been shown to be more beneficial for some chemotherapeutic agents that require a higher pH to work appropriately.

Can Help You Maintain a Healthy Weight

Although the diet isn't solely focused on fat loss, following an alkaline diet meal plan for weight loss can certainly help protect against obesity.

Limiting consumption of acid-forming foods and eating more alkaline-forming foods may make it easier to lose weight due to the diet's ability to decrease leptin levels and inflammation. This affects both your hunger and fat-burning abilities.

Since alkaline-forming foods are anti-inflammatory foods, consuming an alkaline diet gives your body a chance to achieve normal leptin levels and feel satisfied from eating the amount of calories you really need.

If weight loss is one of your main goals, one of the best approaches to try is a keto alkaline diet, which is low in carbs and high in healthy fats.

How to Follow

How do you keep your body alkaline? Here are some key tips for following an alkaline diet:

Buy Organic Alkaline Foods

Experts feel that one important consideration in regard to eating an alkaline diet is to become knowledgeable about what type of soil your produce was grown in — since fruits and vegetables that are grown in organic, mineral-dense soil tend to be more alkalizing. Research shows that the type of soil that plants are grown in can significantly influence their vitamin and mineral content, which means not all "alkaline foods" are created equally.

The ideal pH of soil for the best overall availability of essential nutrients in plants is between 6 and 7.

Acidic soils below a pH of 6 may have reduced calcium and magnesium, and soil above a pH of 7 may result in chemically unavailable iron, manganese, copper and zinc.

Soil that's well-rotated, organically sustained and exposed to wildlife/grazing cattle tends to be the healthiest.

Eat More Alkaline Foods and a Lot Fewer Acidic Foods

See the list below of the best alkaline diet foods, plus those to avoid.

Drink Alkaline Water

Alkaline water has a pH of 9 to 11. Distilled water is just fine to drink. Water filtered with a reverse osmosis filter is slightly acidic, but it's still a far better option than tap water or purified bottled water.

Adding pH drops, lemon or lime, or baking soda to your water can also boosts its alkalinity. You can also make your own electrolyte drink.

(Optional) Test Your pH Level

If you're curious to know your pH level before implementing the tips below, you can test your pH by purchasing strips at your local health food store or pharmacy. You can measure your pH with saliva or urine.

Your second urination of the morning will give you the best results. You compare the colors on your test strip to a chart that comes with your test strip kit.

During the day, the best time to test your pH is one hour before a meal and two hours after a meal. If you test with your saliva, you want to try to stay between 6.8 and 7.2.

Best Alkaline Foods

Although you don't have to be strict vegetarian to eat a high-alkaline diet, the diet is mostly plant-based. Here is a list of foods to emphasize most:

• Fresh fruits and vegetables promote alkalinity the most. Which are the best choices; for example, are bananas alkaline? What about broccoli? Some of the top picks include mushrooms, citrus, dates, raisins, spinach, grapefruit, tomatoes, avocado, summer black radish, alfalfa grass, barley grass, cucumber, kale, jicama, wheatgrass, broccoli, oregano, garlic, ginger, green beans, endive, cabbage, celery, red beet, watermelon, figs and ripe bananas.

- All raw foods: Ideally try to consume a good portion of your produce raw. Uncooked fruits and vegetables are said to be biogenic or "life-

giving." Cooking foods depletes alkalizing minerals. Increase your intake of raw foods, and try juicing or lightly steaming fruits and vegetables.
- Plant proteins: Almonds, navy beans, lima beans and most other beans are good choices.
- Alkaline water.
- Green drinks: Drinks made from green vegetables and grasses in powder form are loaded with alkaline-forming foods and chlorophyll. Chlorophyll is structurally similar to our own blood and helps alkalize the blood.
- Other foods to eat on an alkaline diet include sprouts, wheatgrass, kamut, fermented soy, like natto or tempeh, and seeds.

Acidic Foods

What foods should you avoid when following an alkaline diet eating plan? Acidic foods such as the following:

- High-sodium foods: Processed foods contain tons of sodium chloride — table salt — which constricts blood vessels and creates acidity.
- Cold cuts and conventional meats
- Processed cereals (such as corn flakes)
- Eggs

- Caffeinated drinks and alcohol
- Oats and whole wheat products: All grains, whole or not, create acidity in the body. Americans ingest most of their plant food quota in the form of processed corn or wheat.
- Milk: Calcium-rich dairy products cause some of the highest rates of osteoporosis. That's because they create acidity in the body! When your bloodstream becomes too acidic, it steals calcium (a more alkaline substance) from the bones to try to balance out the pH level. The best way to prevent osteoporosis is to eat lots of alkaline green leafy veggies!
- Peanuts and walnuts
- Pasta, rice, bread and packaged grain products
- What other kinds of habits can cause acidity in your body? The biggest offenders include:
- Alcohol and drug use
- High caffeine intake
- Antibiotic overuse
- Artificial sweeteners
- Chronic stress
- Declining nutrient levels in foods due to industrial farming
- Low levels of fiber in the diet
- Lack of exercise
- Excess animal meats in the diet (from non-grass-fed sources)

- Excess hormones from foods, health and beauty products, and plastics
- Exposure to chemicals and radiation from household cleansers, building materials, computers, cell phones and microwaves
- Food coloring and preservatives
- Overexercise
- Pesticides and herbicides
- Pollution
- Poor chewing and eating habits
- Processed and refined foods
- Shallow breathing

Vs. Paleo Diet

- The Paleo diet and alkaline diet have many things in common and a lot of the same benefits, such as lowered risk for nutrient deficiencies, reduced inflammation levels, better digestion, weight loss or management, and so on.
- Some things that the two have in common include eliminating added sugars, reducing intake of pro-inflammatory omega-6 fatty acids, eliminating grains and processed carbs, decreasing or eliminating dairy/milk intake, and increasing intake of fruits and veggies.
- However, there are several important things to consider if you plan to follow the Paleo diet.

The Paleo diet eliminates all dairy products, including yogurt and kefir, which can be valuable sources of probiotics and minerals for many people — plus the Paleo diet doesn't always emphasize eating organic foods or grass-fed/free-range meat (and in moderation/limited quantities).

- Additionally, the Paleo diet tends to include lots of meat, pork and shellfish, which have their own drawbacks.
- Eating too many animal sources of protein in general can actually contribute to acidity, not alkalinity. Beef, chicken, cold cuts, shellfish and pork can contribute to sulfuric acid buildup in the blood as amino acids are broken down. Try to obtain the best quality animal products you can, and vary your intake of protein foods to balance your pH level best.

The basic premise of the alkaline diet is to eat foods ranking high on the pH list and fall within the acceptable ranges for protein, fat, and carbs. You don't need to follow any specific foods or eat a certain times; you simply need to eat foods that tip your pH balance into alkaline levels.

Fruits

Not all fruits are on the approved list, however, you may eat:

- Apples
- Apricots
- Black currants
- Lemon juice
- Oranges
- Peaches
- Pears
- Vegetables
- Not all vegetables are on the approved list, however, you may eat:
- Asparagus
- Broccoli
- Carrots
- Celery
- Cucumber
- Green beans
- Beverages

You can drink alcohol and coffee in moderation on this diet:

- Coffee, which is slightly acid
- Red and white wine

The alkaline diet promotes an increased intake of fruits and vegetables while discouraging heavily processed foods that are high in sodium and saturated fat, and even some healthy foods.

Proteins

- Red meat
- Poultry
- Fish
- Carbohydrates
- Muffins
- Doughnuts
- Cereal
- Crackers
- Grains
- Potatoes

How to Prepare the Alkaline Diet & Tips

The alkaline diet allows consumption of certain foods recommended by the United States Department of Agriculture (USDA), and recommends limiting legumes, any red meat, eggs, and dairy. The diet can fall within accepted ranges for the amount of protein, carbs, fat, and other nutrients, but is not backed by any science.2

Because of the amount of fresh produce you can eat, you do not need to cook any special entrees or meals. But, the alkaline diet restrictive and advises you to stay away from hard alcohol, soda, sweetened juice, artificial sweeteners, nuts, legumes, dairy, eggs, grains, and beans.

Sample Shopping List

The alkaline diet does not require fasting. The idea behind the alkaline diet is to eat more alkaline foods and fewer acidic foods. This is not a definitive shopping list and if following the diet, you may find other foods that work best for you.

- Extra Virgin Olive Oil
- Fruits (apples, berries and melon)
- Vegetables (spinach, broccoli, etc)
- Coffee
- Dark Leafy Greens (kale, Swiss chard, etc)
- Avocado oil

Sample Meal Plan

The alkaline diet allows all of the foods recommended by the USDA to be consumed, although it restricts certain amounts of grains, legumes, animal protein, and dairy, and therefore is not necessarily considered healthy as it may lack varied nutrients and balance. This is not an all-inclusive meal plan and if following the diet, you may find other meals that work best for you.

Day 1

- Breakfast: Apples and cinnamon
- Lunch: Garden salad with roasted vegetables, topped with a squeeze of lemon
- Dinner: Sweet potato and sautéed spinach

Day 2

- Breakfast: Fruit smoothie
- Lunch: Steamed asparagus and spinach salad
- Dinner: Spiralized carrots with marinara sauce with sauteed mushrooms

Day 3

- Breakfast: Pears, peaches, and coffee
- Lunch: Vegetable hummus with carrots, celery, and grape tomatoes
- Dinner: Grilled mushrooms, peppers, and onions with mild salsaan

Is the Alkaline Diet a Healthy Choice for You?

Requiring little meal planning and easy grocery shopping, the alkaline diet emphasizes loads of fruits and vegetables with limited to no amounts of processed foods, starches, and red meat.

If you prefer a variety of foods in your diet and cannot remove meat, the alkaline diet could be challenging. In addition, a number of foods that are considered high in acid, such as whole grains, beans, and nuts, are actually nutritious and should be included in a balanced diet, according to the USDA.

Chapter two

Recipes for alkaline diet

Garden Pasta Salad

A zesty garden pasta salad with lots of crunchy vegetables tossed in Italian dressing.

Prep Time: 25 mins

Cook Time: 15 mins

Additional Time: 1 hr

Total Time: 1 hr 40 mins

Servings: 10

Ingredients

1 (16 ounce) package tri-color rotini pasta

2 large tomatoes, diced

2 stalks celery, chopped

½ cup thinly sliced carrots

½ cup chopped green bell pepper

½ cup cucumber, peeled and thinly sliced

¼ cup chopped onion

1 ½ (16 ounce) bottles Italian-style salad dressing, or to taste

½ cup grated Parmesan cheese

Directions

Mix tomatoes, celery, carrots, bell pepper, cucumber, and onion together in a large bowl. Add cooled pasta, salad dressing, and Parmesan; mix until well combined. Cover and chill for 1 hour before serving.

Bring a large pot of lightly salted water to a boil; cook pasta at a boil until tender yet firm to the bite, about 8 minutes. Rinse under cold water, and drain.

Nutrition Facts (per serving)

Calories: 385, Fat: 21g, Carbs: 43g, Protein: 8g

Copycat Olive Garden Salad

Here's my copycat version of the famous Olive Garden Salad –the secret to your favorite soup, salad, and breadsticks combo–and now you can enjoy it at home anytime.

Prep Time: 15 mins

Stand Time: 5 mins

Total Time: 20 mins

Servings: 8

Ingredients

Dressing:

1/4 cup extra-virgin olive oil

3 tablespoons mayonnaise

1 tablespoon white wine vinegar

1 tablespoon fresh lemon juice

1 1/2 teaspoons white sugar

1 teaspoon kosher salt

3/4 teaspoon freshly ground black pepper

1/2 teaspoon Italian seasoning

1 garlic clove, crushed

1/4 cup freshly grated Parmesan cheese

Salad:

2 (5 ounce) packages American salad mix

3/4 cup pitted black olives

3/4 cup pickled pepperoncini

1/2 cup thinly sliced red onion

2 plum tomatoes, sliced

1 (4 1/2 ounce) package large seasoned croutons

Directions

Combine olive oil, mayonnaise, vinegar, lemon juice, sugar, salt, pepper, Italian seasoning, garlic, and Parmesan in a food processor, and process until thoroughly combined.

Combine salad mix, olives, pepperoncini, onion, tomatoes, and croutons in a large bowl. Drizzle salad with dressing; toss to coat. Let stand for 5 minutes before serving.

overhead view of bowl of mixed Italian salad with wooden salad spoons

Nutrition Facts (per serving)

156 Calories, 13g Fat, 8g Carbs, 2g Protein

Russian Garden Salad

This delicious Russian garden salad is one of the most popular and traditional salads in Russia.

Prep Time: 20 mins

Total Time: 20 mins

Servings: 4

Yield: 4 servings

Ingredients

10 romaine lettuce leaves, chopped

4 tomatoes, chopped

1 large cucumber, sliced

1 onion, sliced

½ cup fresh parsley, chopped

1 tablespoon salt

2 tablespoons lemon juice

1 tablespoon extra-virgin olive oil

1 cup sour cream

Directions

Toss the romaine lettuce, tomatoes, cucumber, onion, and parsley together in a large bowl; season with salt. Drizzle the lemon juice and olive oil over the salad; stir. Add the sour cream and mix until evenly coated.

Shrimp Garden Salad

This is my version of a simple garden salad which I changed by adding a small tin of shrimp.

Prep Time: 15 mins

Total Time: 15 mins

Servings: 6

Yield: 6 servings

Ingredients

1 head romaine lettuce- rinsed, dried and chopped

2 bunches radishes, sliced

1 bunch green onions, chopped

1 cucumber, cleaned and chopped

3 tomatoes, chopped

3 stalks celery, chopped

1 (4.5 ounce) can small shrimp, drained

Directions

In a large bowl, combine the Romaine, radishes, green onions, cucumber, tomatoes, celery and shrimp. Toss with favorite salad dressing and serve.

Nutrition Facts (per serving)

73 Calories, 1g Fat, 10g Carbs, 8g Protein

Edamame (green soybeans), corn, black beans, and garden-fresh cherry tomatoes are tossed in a cilantro-lime vinaigrette in this colorful salad that makes a nice addition to any meal.

Prep Time: 15 mins

Cook Time: 10 mins

Additional Time: 2 hrs

Total Time: 2 hrs 25 mins

Servings: 8

Ingredients

Vinaigrette:

⅓ cup chopped fresh cilantro

5 tablespoons red wine vinegar

3 tablespoons grapeseed oil

2 medium limes, juiced

2 cloves garlic, minced

1 teaspoon white sugar

¾ teaspoon salt

Salad:

1 (1 pound) package frozen shelled edamame (green soybeans)

3 cups frozen corn kernels

1 (15 ounce) can black beans, rinsed and drained

1 pint cherry tomatoes, quartered

4 green onions, thinly sliced

Directions

Make the vinaigrette: Whisk cilantro, vinegar, oil, lime juice, garlic, sugar, and salt together in a large bowl until well combined.

Make the salad: Bring a large pot of lightly salted water to a boil. Add edamame and cook for 3 minutes. Add corn and cook for 1 more minute. Drain very well.

Pour edamame and corn into the large bowl with vinaigrette, then add beans, cherry tomatoes, and green onions; gently mix until all ingredients are coated. Cover and refrigerate until flavors have blended, at least 2 hours.

Creamy Garden Cucumber Salad

Wonderful ranch cucumber salad side dish to have at your family cookouts! Quick and easy, and the flavors really transform your garden cucumbers. You can also add grape or cherry tomatoes for enhancement. Keep in the refrigerator until ready to serve.

Prep Time: 15 mins

Additional Time: 3 hrs

Total Time: 3 hrs 15 mins

Servings: 8

Ingredients

4 large cucumbers, sliced

salt and ground black pepper to taste

½ cup half-and-half

½ cup sour cream

½ cup mayonnaise

5 large green onions, thinly sliced

1 (1 ounce) package ranch dressing mix (such as Lipton® Recipe Secrets®)

1 ½ tablespoons white sugar

1 tablespoon dried dill weed

1 teaspoon celery salt

2 teaspoons lime juice

Directions

Layer cucumber slices in a large bowl, generously seasoning each layer of cucumber with salt and pepper. Cover the bowl with plastic wrap and refrigerate for 3 hours.

Drain liquid from cucumbers. Gently press cucumber slices with paper towels to absorb any remaining liquid.

Stir half-and-half, sour cream, mayonnaise, green onions, ranch dressing mix, sugar, dill, celery salt, and lime juice together in a small bowl; pour over cucumber slices and gently stir to coat.

Basic Fruit Smoothie

This is a great fruit smoothie recipe consisting of fruit, fruit juice, and ice. I like to use whatever fresh fruits I crave that day... Berries, mangos, papayas, kiwi fruit, etc. Experiment with your favorites!

Prep Time: 10 mins

Total Time: 10 mins

Servings: 4

Ingredients

1 quart strawberries, hulled

2 fresh peaches - peeled, pitted, and sliced

1 banana, broken into chunks

2 cups ice

1 cup orange-peach-mango juice

Directions

Gather all ingredients.

Overhead shot of the ingredients gathered to make a fruit smoothie

Combine strawberries, peaches, and banana in a blender; blend until smooth.

Overhead shot of a blender with ingredients for a fruit smoothie

Add ice and pour in juice; blend again to desired consistency.

Overhead shot of a blended fruit smoothie in a blender

Enjoy!

Purple Monstrosity Fruit Smoothie

This is a great smoothie for breakfast - and sometimes dinner! You can substitute the orange juice with any mix of juices or even soy milk! The soy milk adds more of a milk shake quality than the juice does.

Prep Time: 5 mins

Total Time: 5 mins

Servings: 5

Yield: 4 to 6 drinks

Ingredients

2 frozen bananas, skins removed and cut in chunks

½ cup frozen blueberries

1 cup orange juice

1 tablespoon honey (Optional)

1 teaspoon vanilla extract (Optional)

Directions

Place bananas, blueberries and juice in a blender, puree. Use honey and/or vanilla to taste. Use more or less liquid depending on the thickness you want for your smoothie.

Nutrition Facts (per serving)

88 Calories, 0g Fat, 21g Carbs, 1g Protein

This yogurt smoothie recipe is delicious! You may substitute the strawberries for any other berries or fruit.

Prep Time: 5 mins

Total Time: 5 mins

Servings: 2

Ingredients

1 cup strawberries

1 banana

½ cup yogurt

¼ cup pineapple juice

1 ½ teaspoons white sugar

1 teaspoon orange juice

1 teaspoon milk

Directions

Gather all ingredients.

Ingredients to make fruit and yogurt smoothies

Combine strawberries, banana, yogurt, pineapple juice, sugar, orange juice, and milk in a blender.

A blender pitcher with strawberries, banana, yogurt, pineapple juice, sugar, orange juice, and milk

Blend until smooth.

A blender with pureed fruit and yogurt

Nutrition Facts (per serving)

146 Calories, 1g Fat, 31g Carbs, 5g Protein

Triple Threat Fruit Smoothie

A wonderful, delightful fruit smoothie...it will help you cool down after a hot day in the sun.

Prep Time: 5 mins

Total Time: 5 mins

Servings: 4

Yield: 4 servings

Ingredients

• 1 kiwi, sliced

• 1 banana, peeled and chopped

• ½ cup blueberries

• 1 cup strawberries

• 1 cup ice cubes

• ½ cup orange juice

• 1 (8 ounce) container peach yogurt

Directions

1. In a blender, blend the kiwi, banana, blueberries, strawberries, ice, orange juice, and yogurt until smooth.

Nutrition Facts (per serving)

135 Calories

1g Fat

30g Carbs

4g Protein

2-Ingredient Frozen Fruit Smoothie

This frozen fruit smoothie has two ingredients and is both refreshing and hydrating. It's a great way to get a tropical chill on a sultry summer day, without any added sweetener.

Prep Time: 5 mins

Cook Time: 0 mins

Total Time: 5 mins

Servings: 1

Yield: 1 smoothie

Ingredients

• 9 ounces frozen mixed fruit (strawberries, peaches, pineapple, and mango)

• 8 ounces coconut water

• 1 blackberry (optional)

• 1 strawberry (optional)

Directions

1. Pour coconut water into a Vitamix blender. Add frozen fruit. Slowly turn the blender to Variable 10, then to High 10. Blend for 45 seconds.

2. Pour smoothie into glass; garnish with strawberry and blackberry if desired.

Cook's Note:

The blender you have will make a difference. The Vitamix is a high powered blender. If you have a standard blender, you'll need to blend for a longer time.

Nutrition Facts (per serving)

161 Calories

1g Fat

38g Carbs

3g Protein

This steamed asparagus is tender and tasty! Try using vinaigrette dressing in place of the butter, too.

Prep Time: 10 mins

Cook Time: 5 mins

Total Time: 15 mins

Servings: 4

Ingredients

• 1 bunch asparagus spears

• 1 teaspoon butter

• ¼ teaspoon salt

Directions

1. Place 3 cups water in the bottom half of a steamer pan set. Add butter and salt and bring to a boil.

2. Trim dry ends off of asparagus. If spears are thick, peel them lightly with a vegetable peeler.

3. Place asparagus spears in the top half of the steamer pan set. Steam until asparagus is tender, 5 to 10 minutes depending on thickness.

Recipe Tip

If you don't have a steamer pan set, you can use a steamer basket inserted into a large pot.

Nutrition Facts (per serving)

32 Calories

1g Fat

4g Carbs

3g Protein

The Best Steamed Asparagus

Steaming asparagus in the microwave is the best way to cook asparagus to enjoy its flavor. It comes out absolutely perfect. For the wine, we recommend Pinot Grigio.

Prep Time: 5 mins

Cook Time: 5 mins

Additional Time: 5 mins

Total Time: 15 mins

Servings: 4

Ingredients

1 pound fresh asparagus spears, trimmed

¼ cup white wine

2 tablespoons butter

Directions

Place asparagus in a microwave-safe dish. Pour in wine and dot with butter.

Cover loosely and cook in the microwave on high until bright green and tender, about 3 minutes. Allow to stand for 5 minutes before serving.

Nutrition Facts (per serving)

86 Calories, 6g Fat, 5g Carbs, 3g Protein

Mena's Simple Steamed Asparagus

This is a quick and easy way to prepare a steamed asparagus side dish in the microwave.

Prep Time: 5 mins

Cook Time: 5 mins

Additional Time: 5 mins

Total Time: 15 mins

Servings: 4

Yield: 4 servings

Ingredients

1 bunch fresh asparagus

¼ cup water

1 lemon

⅛ teaspoon ground black pepper

⅛ teaspoon garlic powder (Optional)

Directions

Take each spear of asparagus and break it towards the end, wherever it naturally snaps, to remove woody ends. Place asparagus in a microwave-safe glass container with a lid. Pour in water.

Roll lemon on a flat work surface to release the juices; slice in half. Squeeze each half over the asparagus. Sprinkle with pepper and garlic powder.

Cover container and place in the microwave. Cook on high until tender-crisp, 5 to 6 minutes. Drain and let stand for 5 minutes before serving.

Nutrition Facts (per serving)

29 Calories, 0g Fat, 7g Carbs, 3g Protein

This asparagus quiche has a delectable combination of tender asparagus, crisp bacon pieces, and Swiss cheese for a tasty brunch, lunch, or dinner.

Prep Time: 20 mins

Cook Time: 50 mins

Total Time: 1 hr 10 mins

Servings: 12

Yield: 2 (8-inch) quiches

Ingredients

1 pound fresh asparagus, trimmed and cut into ½-inch pieces

10 slices bacon

2 (8-inch) unbaked pie shells

1 egg white, lightly beaten

2 cups shredded Swiss cheese

4 large eggs

1 ½ cups half-and-half cream

¼ teaspoon ground nutmeg

salt and pepper to taste

Directions

Preheat the oven to 400 degrees F (200 degrees C).

Place asparagus in a steamer over 1 inch boiling water. Cover and cook until tender but still firm, 2 to 6 minutes. Drain and cool.

Place bacon in a large skillet and cook over medium-high heat, turning occasionally, until evenly browned, about 10 minutes. Drain bacon slices on paper towels. Crumble and set aside.

Brush pie shells with beaten egg white. Sprinkle crumbled bacon and steamed asparagus into pie shells. Sprinkle Swiss cheese over bacon and asparagus.

Beat eggs, half-and-half, nutmeg, salt, and pepper in a bowl until well combined. Pour egg mixture on top of cheese.

Bake uncovered in the preheated oven until filling is set, 35 to 40 minutes. Let cool to room temperature before serving.

Nutrition Facts (per serving)

384 Calories, 25g Fat, 26g Carbs, 15g Protein

This is a very elegant and easy side dish to serve for a special occasion.

Prep Time: 10 mins

Cook Time: 10 mins

Total Time: 20 mins

Servings: 6

Yield: 6 servings

Ingredients

1 bunch asparagus spears, ends trimmed

2 tablespoons butter

1 (8 ounce) package sliced mushrooms

1 onion, minced

½ cup coarsely chopped pecans

½ teaspoon garlic powder

½ teaspoon dried basil

¼ teaspoon salt

¼ teaspoon black pepper

½ cup freshly grated Parmesan cheese

Directions

Steam the asparagus spears in a basket-style steamer over boiling water until tender, 5 to 10 minutes. Drain and remove to a serving dish; keep warm.

Meanwhile, melt half of the butter in a large skillet over medium-high heat. Once melted (it's ok if it begins to brown), stir in the sliced mushrooms, and cook until they brown, soften, and begin to release their liquid; pour into a serving dish, and set aside. Melt the remaining butter in the skillet, and stir in the onions. Cook until the onions soften and turn translucent, about 3 minutes. Season with garlic powder, basil, salt and pepper. Stir in the chopped pecans, and cook for a minute more.

Sprinkle the onion mixture with half of the Parmesan cheese, and stir in the reserved mushrooms. Pour over the asparagus in the serving dish and sprinkle with remaining cheese.

Nutrition Facts (per serving)

170 Calories, 14g Fat, 8g Carbs, 7g Protein

Spring Herb Hummus Vegetable Garden

Vegetable platters need not look all look the same. Here, fresh spring vegetables sit in an herb-laced hummus to resemble a spring garden in full bloom.

My kids loved plucking the crisp vegetables from the garden, so much so that I think they forgot that they were filling themselves up with such a healthful snack.

Prep Time: 20 mins

Total Time: 20 mins

Servings: 6

Yield: 6 servings

Ingredients

2 (15 ounce) cans chickpeas (garbanzo beans), drained and rinsed

½ cup tahini

½ cup water

1 lemon, zested and juiced

¼ cup chopped fresh basil

¼ cup chopped fresh parsley

¼ cup chopped fresh chives

¼ cup chopped fresh mint

1 clove garlic, peeled

½ teaspoon salt

6 small carrots with greens still attached, or as desired

6 sugar snap peas, or as desired

6 fresh asparagus, or as desired

6 radishes with greens, halved, or as desired

6 small stalks celery hearts with leaves, or as desired

Directions

Blend chickpeas, tahini, water, lemon zest, lemon juice, basil, parsley, chives, mint, garlic, and salt in a blender until smooth. Spread hummus in a 2-inch deep baking dish.

Arrange carrots, sugar snap peas, asparagus, radishes, and celery in neat rows in the hummus to resemble a garden.

Cook's Note:

Feel free to use your favorite dip here just so long as it's thick enough to help the vegetables stand. It should be at least 1-inch thick in the pan to support the vegetables.

Taste hummus after blending and add more salt or lemon juice, if you'd like.

Use any variety of fresh herbs in place of the ones listed here.

Use fresh vegetables of varying heights, textures and color. My favorites are slender carrots with a bit of their greens still attached, snap peas, radishes cut in half with their greens, asparagus tops (great raw or you can blanch if you'd like), celery (the interior stalks with the leaves are my favorite), and small peppers.

Nutrition Facts (per serving)

304 Calories, 12g Fat, 41g, Carbs, 12g Protein

Hummus Chicken

This is a fast, delicious weeknight dinner. Use any flavor of hummus that you prefer, but spicy works well for me. Serve with a side of rice.

Prep Time: 10 mins

Cook Time: 35 mins

Total Time: 45 mins

Servings: 2

Yield: 2 servings

Ingredients

1 green bell pepper, chopped

1 onion, chopped

2 tablespoons olive oil

2 skinless, boneless chicken breast halves

½ cup prepared hummus

½ lemon, juiced

1 teaspoon paprika

Directions

Preheat an oven to 450 degrees F (230 degrees C).

Stir green bell pepper and onion together in the bottom of a 9-inch casserole dish. Drizzle olive oil over the vegetables; stir to coat.

Coat chicken breasts completely with a thin layer of hummus and place atop the vegetables. Drizzle lemon juice over the chicken and dust with paprika.

Cook chicken breasts in the preheated oven until no longer pink in the center and the juices run clear, about 35 minutes. An instant-read thermometer inserted into the center should read at least 165 degrees F (74 degrees C).

Nutrition Facts (per serving)

404 Calories, 22g Fat, 25g Carbs, 30g Protein

I tinkered a bit with what I found in other recipes and this is the result. I think I like my results. I stirred in a small handful of tamari-flavored pumpkin seeds just before serving (couldn't find plain ones) and sprinkled a bit of paprika on top to make it look nice.

Prep Time: 15 mins

Additional Time: 2 hrs

Total Time: 2 hrs 15 mins

Servings: 16

Yield: 16 servings

Ingredients

2 tablespoons lemon juice

2 tablespoons tahini

3 cloves garlic

¾ teaspoon salt

2 (15 ounce) cans garbanzo beans, drained

2 teaspoons extra-virgin olive oil

1 (15 ounce) can pumpkin puree

1 teaspoon ground cumin

½ teaspoon cayenne pepper

¼ cup toasted pumpkin seed kernels, or more to taste

1 pinch paprika

Directions

Pulse lemon juice, tahini, garlic, and salt together in a food processor or blender until smooth. Add garbanzo beans and olive oil and pulse until smooth. Add pumpkin, cumin, and cayenne pepper; process until well blended. Transfer hummus to a container with a lid and refrigerate at least 2 hours.

Fold pumpkin seeds into hummus; garnish with paprika.

Grilled Portobello Mushrooms

Grilled portobello mushrooms are the steaks of the mushroom family. Here they're marinated and grilled for a yummy vegan appetizer or summer side dish!

Prep Time: 10 mins

Cook Time: 10 mins

Additional Time: 1 hr

Total Time: 1 hr 20 mins

Servings: 3

Ingredients

3 large portobello mushrooms

¼ cup canola oil

¼ cup balsamic vinegar, or to taste

3 tablespoons chopped onion

4 cloves garlic, minced

Directions

Clean mushrooms; remove stems, reserving them for another use. Place mushroom caps gill-side up in a shallow dish.

Combine oil, balsamic vinegar, onion, and garlic in a small bowl. Pour mixture evenly over mushroom caps; let marinate at room temperature for 1 hour.

Preheat the grill to medium-high heat; grease the grate.

Grill over the hot grill until caramelized and tender, about 5 minutes per side; serve warm.

Grilled Stuffed Portobello Mushroom Caps

Grilled portobello mushroom caps, stuffed with a creamy herb and garlic sauce, grape tomatoes, and cheese, make a delicious main course and can be served atop torn salad greens for a complete meal.

Prep Time: 25 mins

Cook Time: 10 mins

Total Time: 35 mins

Servings: 4

Yield: 4 stuffed mushrooms

Ingredients

4 large portobello mushrooms

2 teaspoons olive oil

½ cup PHILADELPHIA Herb & Garlic Cooking Creme

½ cup grape tomatoes, quartered

2 tablespoons Kraft 100% Parmesan Shredded Cheese

1 green onion, thinly sliced

Directions

Preheat the grill to medium heat and grease the grates. Line a baking sheet with aluminum foil.

Discard stems from mushrooms; scrape out gills with a small spoon. Brush mushrooms with oil.

Cook mushrooms on the preheated grill until slightly softened, about 2 minutes per side. Place mushrooms, rounded-sides down, on the prepared baking sheet. Dab insides of mushroom caps with paper towels to remove excess moisture.

Fill caps with cooking creme, tomatoes, Parmesan cheese, and green onion.

Place the tray with stuffed mushrooms on the grill. Cover and cook until filling is heated through, 6 to 8 minutes. Serve warm.

Grilled Stuffed Portobello Mushrooms

A good dish that goes with almost anything year round. You can double this recipe and serve as a main dish with rice. Enjoy!

Prep Time: 15 mins

Cook Time: 20 mins

Total Time: 35 mins

Servings: 4

Ingredients

½ cup finely chopped red bell pepper

1 clove garlic, minced

¼ cup olive oil

¼ teaspoon onion powder

1 teaspoon salt

½ teaspoon ground black pepper

4 portobello mushroom caps

Directions

Preheat grill for medium heat.

In a large bowl, mix the red bell pepper, garlic, oil, onion powder, salt, and ground black pepper. Spread mixture over gill side of the mushroom caps.

Lightly oil the grill grate. Place mushrooms over indirect heat, cover, and cook for 15 to 20 minutes.

Editor's Note:

This recipe appeared in Allrecipes Magazine and was modified to include fresh thyme.

Portobello Mushroom Burgers

Portobello mushroom burgers are the steak of veggie burgers. Serve these on buns with lettuce, tomato, and aioli sauce. Oh yeah!

Prep Time: 5 mins

Cook Time: 15 mins

Additional Time: 15 mins

Total Time: 35 mins

Servings: 4

Ingredients

4 portobello mushroom caps

¼ cup balsamic vinegar

2 tablespoons olive oil

1 tablespoon minced garlic

1 teaspoon dried basil

1 teaspoon dried oregano

salt and pepper to taste

4 (1 ounce) slices provolone cheese

Directions

Gather all ingredients.

Ingredients to make portobello mushroom burgers

Place mushroom caps, smooth side up, in a shallow dish.

A shallow dish with four portobello mushroom caps

Whisk together balsamic, oil, garlic, basil, and oregano in a small bowl. Season with salt and pepper.

Pour vinaigrette over mushrooms. Let stand at room temperature for 15 minutes or so, turning twice. Preheat grill for medium-high heat.

Brush grill grates with oil. Place mushrooms on grill, reserving marinade for basting.

Grill until just tender, 5 to 8 minutes per side, brushing with marinade frequently.

Top mushrooms with cheese.

Continue grilling until cheese is melted, about 2 minutes.

Serve and enjoy with your choice of toppings.

Note

The nutrition data for this recipe includes information for the full amount of the marinade ingredients. Depending on marinating time, ingredients, cooking method, etc., the actual amount of the marinade consumed will vary.

Gourmet Mushroom Risotto

This mushroom risotto is cooked the slow and painful way, but-oh so worth it. Complements grilled meats and chicken dishes very well. Check the rice by biting into it. It should be slightly al dente (or resist slightly to the tooth but not be hard in the center).

Prep Time: 20 mins

Cook Time: 25 mins

Total Time: 45 mins

Servings: 6

Risotto ranks right up there as one of the greatest dishes you can make with rice. Originating in Italy, risotto is a recipe made by simmering a starchy variety of rice in broth, with flavor-boosting ingredients added like onions, garlic, vegetables, meats, spices, herbs, and cheese. This 5-star recipe for mushroom risotto has thousands of ratings and reviews, and is a top-rated favorite for our Allrecipes community of home cooks.

There are all kinds of tasty add-ins to risotto, and mushrooms are just one of them. Mushrooms add an earthy, savory flavor to risotto that makes it a good complement to main dishes like roast chicken, pork, or beef. You can serve mushroom risotto as a side dish, a main dish, or a starter to a multi-course Italian menu.

Ingredients for Mushroom Risotto

These are the ingredients you'll need to make this mushroom risotto recipe:

Broth: Homemade chicken broth is always the best choice for flavor, but you can use store-bought chicken broth for convenience. Choose low-sodium broth and adjust the seasonings at the end. Since you'll keep it hot on the stove while you're stirring it into the risotto, you can bump up the flavor of the broth by simmering it with scraps of shallots, chives, and mushroom stems left over from prepping the risotto ingredients. To make this vegetarian, substitute vegetable broth.

Olive oil: For sautéing the mushrooms and shallots. You won't be cooking at high heat, so it's okay to use extra virgin olive oil.

Mushrooms: This recipe uses a combination of portobello and white mushrooms. See how to clean mushrooms.

Shallots: If you don't have shallots, you can substitute finely chopped yellow onion.

Rice: To get that signature creamy risotto texture, you must use a particular type of short-grain, high-starch rice like Arborio, Carnaroli, or Vialone Nano that releases its starch as you cook and stir. No other rice will give you the same results.

Wine: The first liquid you add to the pan after you sauté the rice is a half cup of white wine — it will absorb into every grain and create an essential layer of flavor. Choose wisely. Go for a crisp, dry white wine like pinot grigio or sauvignon blanc. If you don't want to use wine, just start with the broth.

Butter: A generous amount of butter at the end adds more creamy texture and rich flavor.

Parmesan cheese: You've come this far. Don't shortchange the flavor of your risotto by using anything other than freshly grated Parmesan cheese.

Chives: Chives cut through the richness and add visual appeal, too. If you don't have chives, fresh parsley is a good substitute.

How to Make Mushroom Risotto

You'll find the measurements and step-by-step recipe directions below, but here are top tips to make the best mushroom risotto:

Hot broth: Keep the broth hot the whole way through. Measure out a little more into the broth pot than the recipe says to make up for evaporation as it sits.

Toast the rice: An essential step to making risotto is to toast the grains in hot oil until they start to turn translucent around the edges. This could take a couple of minutes. Stir continuously during this process.

Stir, stir, stir: Yes, you stir risotto as it simmers. That's what helps release the starch from the grains of rice to make that creamy texture you want. Do you have to stir constantly? No. Stir after each half cup of broth you add to make sure the broth is distributed evenly, then stir again every 30 seconds or so until almost all the broth is absorbed. Add another half cup of broth and repeat. Listen to music. Sip some wine. Good risotto is worth the time it takes.

Low and slow: Keep the broth hot and the risotto at a low simmer throughout.

The perfect texture: Risotto is done when the rice is al dente: firm but not crunchy when you bite into it. It should not be as dry as steamed rice, but should have enough liquid to make it loose. Add just a touch more broth if needed before stirring in the butter and Parmesan cheese.

Serve immediately: Risotto waits for no one. It will continue to cook as it sits even when it's off the heat, so be prepared to dish it up right away.

How to Store Mushroom Risotto

Store leftover risotto in an airtight container in the refrigerator for up to three days. You can reheat risotto, but it won't have the same creamy texture as freshly made risotto. Try forming leftover risotto into patties using an egg and fine breadcrumbs as a binder, and fry them in oil to make risotto cakes.

Can You Freeze Mushroom Risotto?

You can freeze mushroom risotto in an airtight container for up to three month, but the texture won't be the same as freshly made. Use a freezer-safe zip-top bag with the air squeezed out of it. Thaw overnight in the fridge.

Ingredients

6 cups chicken broth, or as needed

3 tablespoons olive oil, divided

1 pound portobello mushrooms, thinly sliced

1 pound white mushrooms, thinly sliced

2 medium shallots, diced

1 ½ cups Arborio rice

½ cup dry white wine

4 tablespoons butter

3 tablespoons finely chopped chives

⅓ cup freshly grated Parmesan cheese

sea salt and freshly ground black pepper to taste

Directions

Gather all ingredients.

Warm broth in a saucepan over low heat.

Meanwhile, warm 2 tablespoons olive oil in a large saucepan over medium-high heat. Add portobello and white mushrooms; cook and stir until soft, about 3 minutes. Remove mushrooms and their liquid to a bowl; set aside.

Add remaining 1 tablespoon olive oil to the saucepan. Stir in shallots and cook for 1 minute. Add rice; cook and stir until rice is coated with oil and pale, golden in color, about 2 minutes.

Pour in wine, stirring constantly until wine is fully absorbed. Add 1/2 cup warm broth to the rice, and stir until the broth is absorbed.

Continue adding broth, 1/2 cup at a time, stirring constantly, until the liquid is absorbed and the rice is tender, yet firm to the bite, about 15 to 20 minutes.

Remove from heat. Stir in reserved mushrooms and their liquid, butter, chives, and Parmesan cheese.

Season with salt and pepper and serve immediately.

Conclusion

Science does not back the alkaline diet. Foods we consume cannot alter our body's pH, which remains tightly regulated on its own. For the average healthy person, your body already monitors its pH levels. What you put into your body will not drastically change this.

Certain health conditions, such as kidney disease and diabetes, can change your pH regulation. However, eating heavy amounts of alkaline foods will not improve your health, and eating acidic foods will not make you more susceptible to disease.

Remember, following a long-term or short-term diet may not be necessary for you and many diets out there simply don't work, especially long-term. While we do not endorse fad diet trends or unsustainable weight loss methods, we present the facts so you can make an informed decision that works best for your nutritional needs, genetic blueprint, budget, and goals.

If your goal is weight loss, remember that losing weight isn't necessarily the same as being your healthiest self, and there are many other ways to pursue health. Exercise, sleep, and other lifestyle factors also play a major role in your overall health.

The best diet is always the one that is balanced and fits your lifestyle.